"After 34 years of practice, Dr. Angrist has become a New York icon of Healing"

-Bones Rodriguez

I've Got Your
BACK

Your
Toolkit
To
Wellness

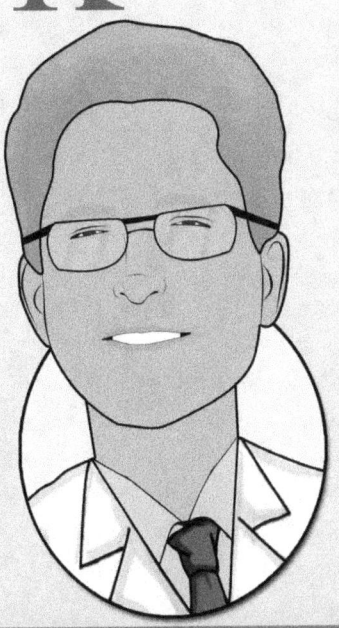

Dr. Arnie Angrist
Wellness Chiropractor

I've Got Your Back
Your Toolkit to Wellness

By Dr. Arnold Angrist
Wellness Chiropractor

http://www.AngristChiro.com

Table of Contents

Acknowledgments

I would like to thank my family, friends, patients and mentors who have given me love and support throughout my life.

I owe the deepest gratitude to my wife Karen and our four boys Matthew, Jason, Benjamin and Jonathan.

I would like to say thank you to my father and mother-in-law, Lester and Marilyn Bornstein as well as my brother and sister-in-law Michael and Sally Oren and Fred and Aura Kuperberg.

Thank you for believing in my alternative approach to health and wellness.

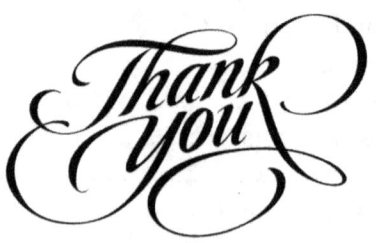

Forward by Bones Rodriguez

I am an actor, author, and entrepreneur born and raised in New York City. I have lived here my entire life, and am always working on something, going somewhere, or meeting someone.

Us New Yorkers are like that.

We face special challenges when it comes to our bodies, and in the hustle and bustle of The City That Never Sleeps, many people are stressed and walking on the concrete can take its toll on your knees and back.

There is high pollution from the many cars and buses, and the overall "rush, rush" energy can really sap you of your energy.

How do you healthfully renew the energy you need to keep up with that kind of pace?

Dr. Angrist has noticed over his 34 years of practice in New York City that many of his patients suffer from stress-related conditions and the wear and tear of New York life. He likes his office to be a special retreat from the outside, where you can get alignment; not just spinal alignment, but a place where you can get your mind, body, and spirit aligned in a healthful way.

So many people sacrifice their health for their monetary gain by staying late at work, or by being stressed over deadlines and goals. Many people sleep terribly because they are so worried about upcoming projects and the next day's work.

After chatting with many chiropractors in other parts of the country, Dr. Angrist realized that so many of his counterparts' patients didn't face the same challenges as his patients in NYC.

That's when he really started to delve into the whole-life philosophy: not only attending to his patients' bodies, but also to their minds and spirits.

New York also has a fantastic energy of excitement and achievement; People here seem to have a different kind of happiness and some can even enjoy the pressure. All you have to do is notice how people handle rush hour when the trains are packed full.

Some people deal with it as just another part of the day, while others constantly feel pressured to fight for extra space, or for a seat, or just breathing room.

You can see it on their faces.

The mental state of the average New Yorker is on high alert, so when Dr. Angrist approaches a patient, he likes to find out about the other parts of their lives aside from their bodies.

Many patients come to see a chiropractor expecting to just "get their backs cracked", but Dr. Angrist likes to see what the causes of the stressors are, and deal with them in a preventative fashion.

Since seeing Dr. Angrist, I find myself more relaxed, flexible and energetic. That back-flipping-but-landing-on-my-neck-injury I suffered from 12 years ago didn't start bothering me until 10 years later, and now it doesn't bother me much anymore. The bi-weekly visits to his office are always a pleasure, and I look forward to them.

I have felt so much better since seeing Dr. Angrist, and I was thrilled to help him produce this book. I hope it helps you, and motivates you to visit him and his magic hands!

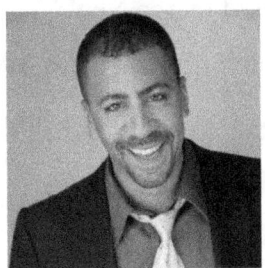

-Bones Rodriguez
http://www.BonesRodriguez.com

About Dr. Angrist

Angrist Chiropractic and Wellness Care has been an established wellness center in New York City and Englewood Cliffs, New Jersey since 1979. Dr. Arnold Angrist D.C., has led this center to fulfill the various health needs and goals of his patients throughout the years. His wellness team consists of chiropractic services, acupuncture, life coaching and nutritional consulting.

Dr. Angrist has been a chiropractor and wellness coach specializing in the harmony of body and mind. He continues to motivate, educate and empower his patients to enjoy a healthy lifestyle. He is known for his personal and holistic approach that ensures that his patients are more accountable for their health by removing interferences in their lives.

He is licensed by the New York and New Jersey state chiropractic associations, a member of the American Chiropractic Association and holds a certificate from the International College of Applied Kinesiology.

Dr. Angrist works with large corporations, teaching employees about posture and stress management. He was the on-call Chiropractor for recording artists at Madison Square Garden.

Yearly he associates with charities such as Dans Music, Smile Forever, Comedy Cures, Teen Impact and City Harvest.

Dr. Angrist enjoys spending time with his family, playing golf and helping his patients move in a direction of wellness. He also has an A+ rating with the Better Business Bureau.

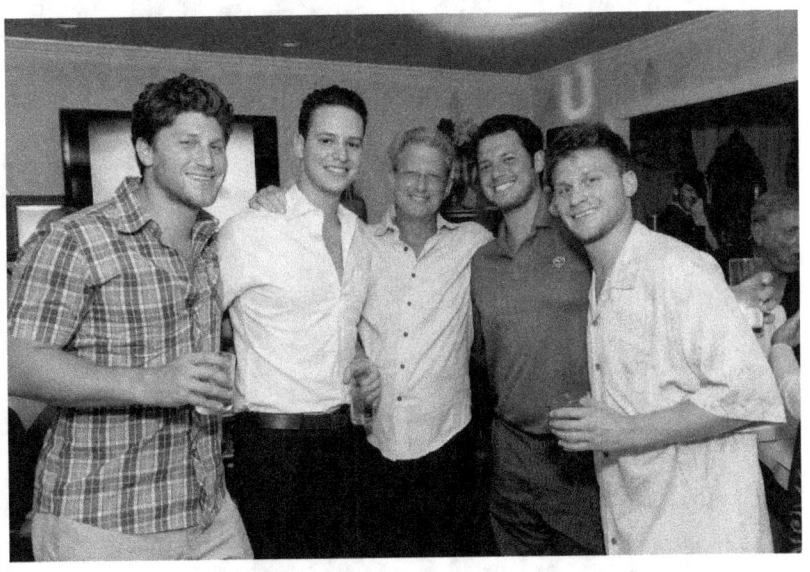

Dr. Angrist and his four sons

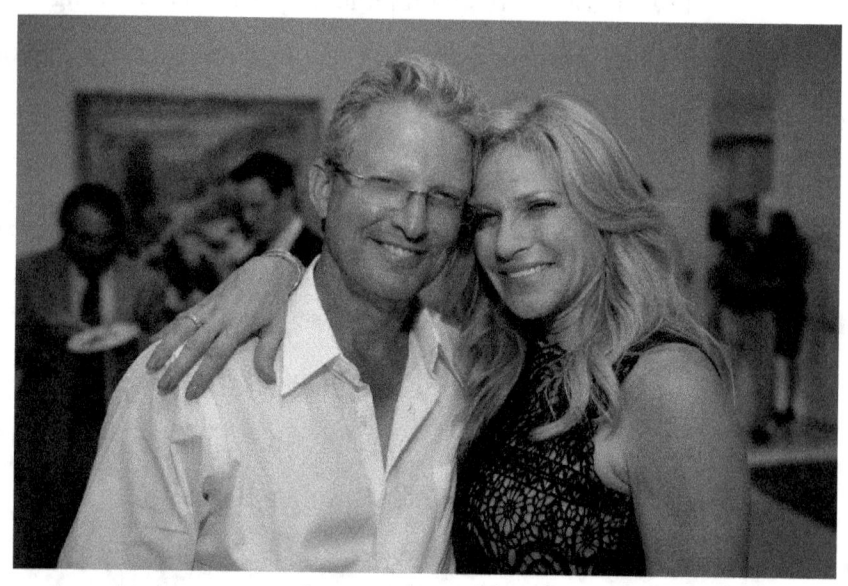

Dr. Angrist and his wife, Karen

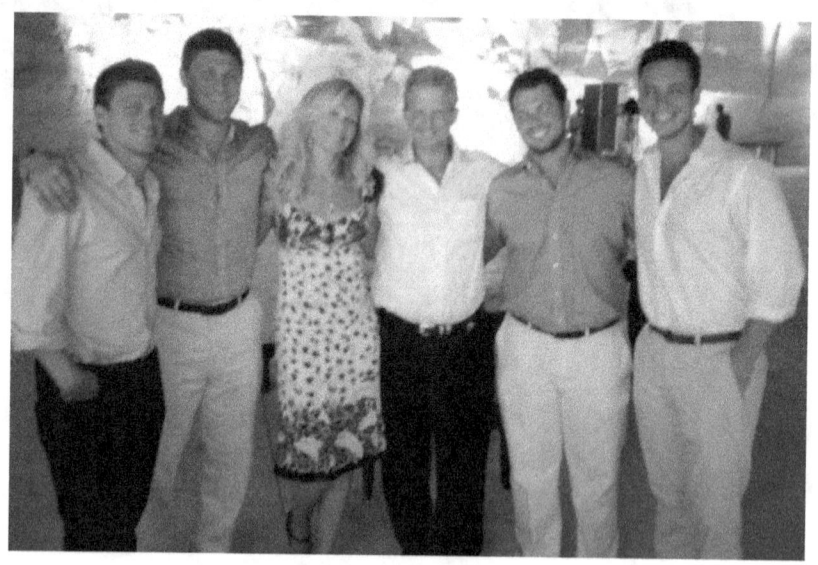

The Angrist Family

Welcome to Angrist Chiropractic and Wellness Care

Welcome to the world of wellness chiropractic. There is a lot of confusion and misunderstanding about what chiropractic is, and about what wellness is. I believe this book will help clarify both of these.

The word "Chiropractic" comes from the Greek words "Cheir and Praxis", meaning practiced or treatment by hand.

"Practiced by hand". (Manual Therapy).

The word wellness has many definitions in our society. My explanation of wellness is that it begins with our state of mind. Wellness is about the health and lifestyle choices we make each and every day. **Here are my five core principals of wellness:**

1. Exercise regularly. Focus on flexibility, core strength.
2. Eat healthy foods daily.
3. Be attentive and conscious of your posture.
4. Try to get 7-9 hours of sleep per night.
5. Have a loving, kind, caring and giving attitude.

These five principals are the foundation for having wellness in our lives. If we can be conscious of these five as well as regularly practicing them, wellness can be attained. The wonderful part is there is no financial cost involved.

The essence of Angrist Chiropractic and Wellness Care combines the manual hands-on approach to enhance flexibility and balance complemented by the five core principals that I ask every patient to apply as best they can in their daily lives.

We will discuss in detail the action steps you need to do to own this wellness lifestyle.

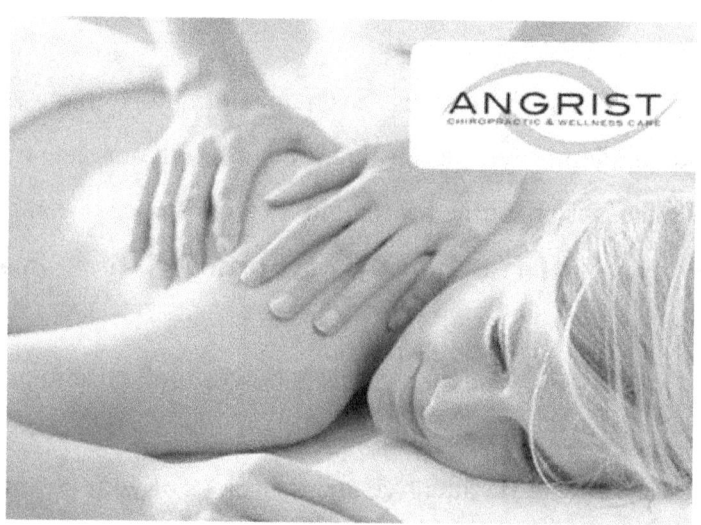

What is Wellness Chiropractic Care?

Wellness chiropractic care consists of a patient receiving a structure of specific wellness concepts, philosophies, and action steps in addition to the actual manual care introduced.

I began my training back in 1976 in Chiropractic school in St. Louis, Missouri as a spinal technician. What that means is that I was able to locate, detect and correct spinal misalignments or subluxations and realign these vertebrae. As a Doctor of Chiropractic (D.C.) I was taught that I was a Doctor of Cause (DC), and the cause was the subluxation or spinal misalignment.

Early in my practice, I always looked for the reason WHY these vertebrae were out of alignment and that determined whether my wellness approach would be effective. There had to be a precursor to that misalignment, because correcting the subluxations didn't seem to be enough.

In order to explain what wellness chiropractic is, I needed to find out WHY the body is out of balance and out of alignment.

Many times patients ask me: "Doc, what is it that I've got?" "What's my diagnosis?" And I say that is a good question, but the key question a patient should ask themselves is WHY am I having this problem?

Any doctor that performs a consultation, evaluation, x-rays, MRI, cat-scans, blood work, etc. can tell you what the diagnosis is. How you decide to treat your condition becomes the vital choice.

We need to get deeper into your lifestyle to understand WHY are you having this problem.

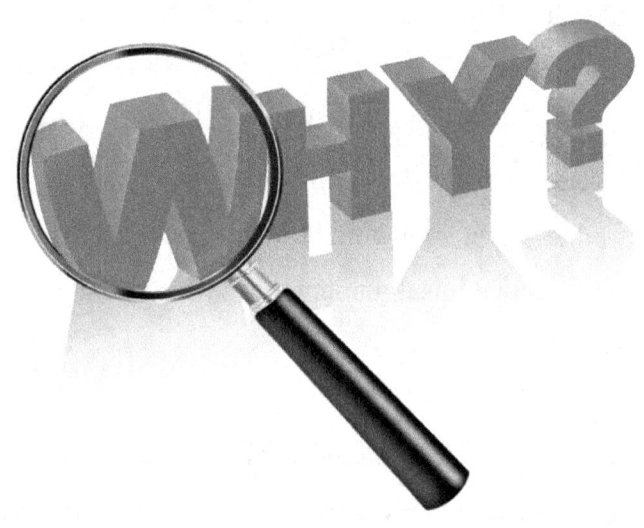

WHY am I having these symptoms?

The WHY is about looking inside yourself for the answer. There is a saying: "if you don't go within, you go without". So let's begin with back pain, a very common complaint in today's society. You can have all of the X-RAYs, MRI's, CAT scans, etc. and any qualified health care provider can diagnose a herniated disc, stenosis, scoliosis, arthritis, etc.

The real question is once you find out the diagnosis, what you are going to do about it? There are four choices: drugs, surgery, therapy or leave it alone. It is a matter of educating the patient of their findings and presenting the optional approaches to apply medically or alternatively.

As I said, once "We know what it is", I now ask my patients, "WHY do you think this happened?" Most patients say they don't have any idea.

If we go back to my five core principals of wellness, I believe the following can help answer the why part of the question:

-When I ask a patient, if she/he has been exercising regularly, stretching the appropriate muscles, doing core strengthening, they usually say no. Well, here is a reason **why** you are having back pain.

-When I ask a patient if she/he has been eating a healthy diet, with lots of fruits, veggies, water, fish, etc. they usually say no. Well, here is another reason **why** you are having back pain. The patient will then tell me that he/she understands that not exercising causes my pain but what does not eating well have to do with my back pain? My response is a healthy diet with fruits, veggies, whole grains, fish and water nourishes and energizes the body while unhealthy foods such as sugars, sodas, caffeine, alcohol and nicotine create toxicity in the body. Within our muscles there is a chemical called lactic acid. We all have it. The problem arises when you have a diet consisting of unhealthy foods which causes a buildup of lactic acid. The more lactic acid, the more stiffness and soreness in our muscles.

-When I ask a patient if she/he has been conscious and aware of their posture, they usually say no. Well, here is another reason **why** you are having back pain. Good posture is essential to creating balance and flexibility to your spine. Posture, in my opinion, is an attitude of standing, walking and being proud. We show patients how to do this in conjunction with the appropriate exercises. Enhancing core strength, (the plank exercise) on a daily basis is an integral part of good posture, complemented by stretching the appropriate muscles.

-When I ask a patient if she/he has been getting enough sleep every night, they usually say no. Well, here is another reason **why** you are having back pain. Getting 7-9 hours of sleep per night recharges and energizes your body and mind for the next day. Sleep heals and enhances the function of your immune system. Did you ever notice when you are sick with a cold, you don't sleep for a few nights. Then finally you get a good night's sleep, how do you feel the next day? Much better. Another key factor for sleep is the position or posture you are in. Are you sleeping on your side, your back, or your stomach? If you sleep on your side or your back you are fine, but if you are a stomach sleeper there is a pretty good chance you will experience back pain at some point. There are two main problems with sleeping on your stomach. Just visualize being on your stomach for six, seven or eight hours and your face being turned to the left or the right. Try walking around like that and see how that feels on your neck and upper back. Pretty uncomfortable. In addition, when you sleep on your stomach, your abdominal muscles don't support your back which causes an increase in the curvature of your lower back (lordosis) which puts added stress and strain on your spinal muscles.

17

-When I ask a patient about their attitude and whether it is loving, kind, caring and giving, they usually reply by asking me how they are supposed to be loving and kind when they are stressed. Well my friends, here is another reason **why** you may be having back pain. Attitude, I believe, may play the biggest role in resolving both the causes and effects of back pain. It may even play the biggest role in resolving many other more serious health related problems. Feelings of anger, resentment, negativity, judgment and fear (which are normal and real), over time can create deep rooted muscular tension. I'm okay with having negative emotions. What I strive for is learning how to not hold on to these negative feelings for a prolonged period of time. In other words, learning to let go.

I will continue to extrapolate on these five core principles throughout this book, but now you have a better feel on how to answer **why** you may be experiencing your pain.

Start reviewing these five areas and see if you can raise the bar. Be more conscious and take the necessary action steps to achieve health and wellness.

WHAT does a Wellness Chiropractor do?

Now we can address the actual manual therapy that is done on a daily basis to help people move in a direction of wellness.

It all starts when a patient calls our office for an appointment. The reason I say this is because I believe the healing begins with a patient's first contact with the staff who manage the front desk. Great customer service and caring from my staff is essential for a patient to begin the process of healing.

Once a patient is in our office they are greeted by my incredible team who help the patient feel at ease. Remember, Chiropractic is an alternative approach where many people are skeptical and afraid. The comforting part is that many of our new patients are referred to us by other patients who have had a rewarding and beneficial experience. Statistics show that only ten percent of Americans have ever been to a Chiropractor. Our job is to explain to patients that have never experienced what we do, that they will leave the office after their first visit with more information and motivation about how they can take better care of their health along with feeling physically better.

At this point the patient is escorted into my office to watch a short five-minute video about who I am and what we do. I then come into my office and sit down with the new patient and talk, not only about their physical problem, but I also try to engage them in the WHY aspect. Once we finish our consultation and I have accepted this patient for care, I proceed to perform a spinal, nerve and muscular evaluation to determine where the imbalances, misalignments, spasms and blockages are.

As I said earlier, chiropractic means practiced by hand. So my evaluation consists of observing posture, assessing core strength and palpating (feeling) the spine and musculature for imbalances.

During the examination and treatment phase I am able to evaluate and treat a patient based on my findings. Many people think that chiropractors are bone doctors because we as a group are known to manipulate, adjust, "crack" or realign the vertebral spinal column.

Moving vertebral bones back into their proper position (chiropractic manipulative therapy) is only one component of what I do. Two additional modalities that I incorporate include soft tissue trigger point massage and physiotherapy.

I believe the sequence of events that causes pain begins with three major stressors in life which adversely affect our muscular and nervous system. These three physical, chemical and emotional stressors cause our muscular system to contract and compress our nervous system. Please see the chart in the Triad of Health chapter.

My primary focus from a manual perspective is to restore balance, strength and flexibility to the spine and its associated soft tissues (muscles, ligaments, tendons, discs and nerves). When this is accomplished via trigger point therapy, physiotherapy and spinal manipulation, vertebrae that were out of position are now realigned.

The muscular component of treatment consists of gentle soft tissue trigger point therapy and myofascial release. This is an unraveling process which is administered manually and releases the tension of the affected muscles. It is very gentle and pain free, even though some trigger points are more sensitive than others. Overall it is a very comfortable experience. We are essentially breaking down the "walls" of tension that have been built up for years.

It is very important to note that each treatment includes a portion of quiet time for the patient. This is what I call "Brain Based Wellness"where both the mind and body relax, which brings you to a state of inner peace.

When your mind relaxes, your nervous system and muscles let go with it, which is an integral part of the healing process.

As we get older, unfortunately, our muscles tend to get tighter rather than looser. Ask yourself if you are tighter or looser than you were twenty years ago? Probably tighter.

I believe we need to understand that tightness, restriction of motion, constriction, congestion, contraction and rigidity of muscles over time plays a vital role in health care today. I think the power of hands-on and manual therapy is enormous for the correction and stabilization of many physical conditions being treated.

The physiotherapy component of the care we provide includes moist hot packs used in conjunction with electrical muscle and nerve stimulation (EMS or TENS). These methods reduce muscle spasm and tightness and increase nerve and blood flow to the affected areas.

If a patient's condition is acute, within 48 hours of the injury or complaint, I utilize ice packs.

After these therapies are applied for ten to twenty-five minutes I re-evaluate the spine and musculature and perform a gentle spinal adjustment (chiropractic manipulative therapy).

This is the essence of what I do when a patient is in our office.

I feel the more tools/techniques we have in our toolkit, the better chance we have to attain great results. Remember the best way for this type of therapy to be effective is what you as the patient do in between your visits. That's your homework. How many tools do you have in your toolkit of health?

Just keep applying the five core principals of wellness.

It's a team effort and I tell every patient, "I need your help. It's not just about you lying on the table and I fix you. I can help you, I can assist you, I can support you, but you have to do the work and begin interrupting some patterns and habits in your life".

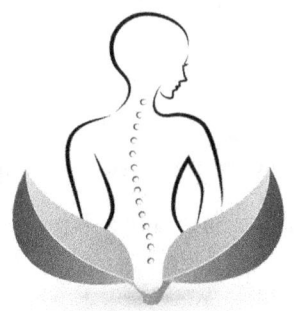

Deepak Chopra, Tony Robbins, and Christopher Reeves

I have a great story that I heard at my friend Tony Robbins' seminar about living in the moment.

Deepak Chopra says the past is history, the future is a mystery, and the present is a gift... that's why it's called the present.

We're a society that tends to live in the past. We're worried about what happened yesterday, and whether the consequences will be positive or negative, but the past is history. It's done.

We tend to worry about tomorrow, and whether the choices we make will lead to something good or bad. But tomorrow is a mystery; we can't really do much about it, except making better choices right now.

Life is really about "Now"; living in the present moment and focusing our attention and our life on it.

I was at a conference with Tony Robbins and he had his friend and guest Christopher Reeves speak and tell his story about the accident that paralyzed him.

Christopher Reeves was riding his horse performing hurdles. There were several jumps in the series, and he was concentrating on the hardest one which was the 7th jump instead of concentrating on the fourth jump (the one he was on) which was actually the easiest jump and that's where his accident occurred.

He took the easy jump for granted. He didn't think about it, he was worrying about the future jumps, the difficult jump instead of focusing on the present, and the easiest jump.

In his own words, he said "If I was thinking about the fourth jump at that time, this never would've happened."

He was injured on something simple because he was not focusing, not being in the present, not living in the moment.

In order to be healthy and well, living in the moment is essential. Our minds can easily get cluttered, and our attention and energy can become so scattered, that we end up living in self – energized turbulence.

What I like to help my patients (and myself!) strive for is inner peace that comes from living in the present moment. As far as I am concerned, inner peace is the highest level of health and wellness we can achieve. Unfortunately, many of us live in the world opposite of inner peace called turbulence (stress). Inner calm, inner peace, tranquility of the mind and body is the ultimate goal.

Being right here, me being with you means not being anywhere else. When you're in the park alone, you're in the park alone. If you are with your spouse or a friend, you're there with them.

Wherever you are, live there in that moment.

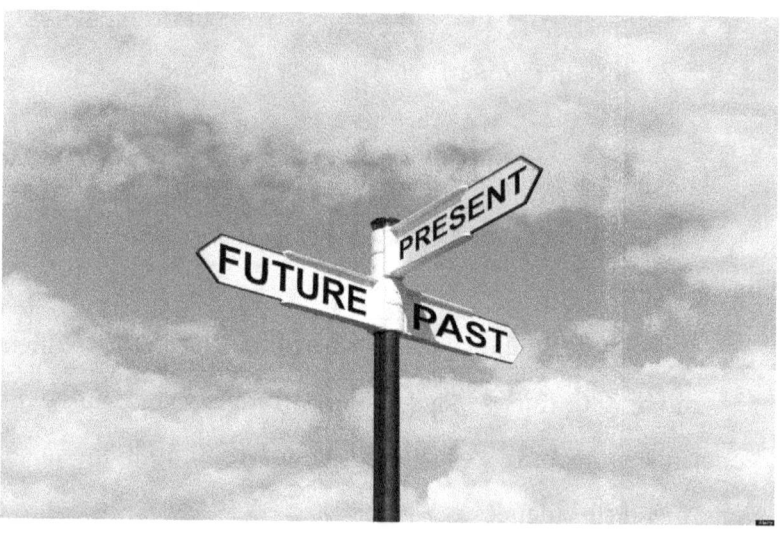

The Bridge between Chiropractic and Wellness

….began for me when I first started in practice. This story allowed me to understand the true connection between chiropractic and wellness.

There was a woman who was a patient of mine, being treated by me, and progressing very well. She said, "I want to refer my husband to you. He has a knee problem and I think you can help him."

I started treating him for about a month or so, and he was doing pretty well. After a month of working on him, she came to me and said, "Thank you so much for helping my husband, but most of all, I want to thank you for the fact that he doesn't abuse me anymore."

I was shocked when I heard this and I realized that what I was trained to do was much bigger than treating any knee or back problem.

It was about changing people's lives. I get goose bumps whenever I tell this story because we all need more inner peace, love and kindness, which eventually show up in our physical body.

Whether it's a back problem or a knee problem, a stomach problem or a headache, together we are able to change that and get amazing results. Regarding this woman, I knew nothing about the terrible situation she was in, but that was a turning point for me understanding what wellness was. I personally get more excited and feel more rewarded when patients tell us that not only do they have less pain, but they've also changed or improved their lives. Remember, alleviating pain is a good start, but changing your life is the ultimate.

The combination of neuromusculoskeletal techniques that I provided helped the husband's knee, but our discussions about letting go, loving and allowing helped him release whatever anger he may have been holding onto. It's my belief that it also helped him transition into being a better person; probably the person his wife fell in love with, and the person who could express himself more freely.

He never said anything about it to me, but the relief I witnessed in her confession spoke volumes to me. My practice was never the same and neither was I.

Clearing up Blockages

After all these years, I still love being a chiropractor, because my goal is to help people improve their lives. This is a never ending process, so it's a never ending activity for me. Some patients call me a healer, but the real healer is you! Healing comes from within you. **The power that made your body, heals your body**. For example if you have a cut it heals on its own. If you have a cold, usually after three or four days your body starts to heal. Even if you break a bone, it heals in about six weeks. Of course, there can be extenuating circumstances, but our bodies have an incredible ability to heal or as I call it, "bouncebackability".

Chiropractic, as well as Acupuncture, Massage, Yoga, Pilates and Meditation focus on finding and removing blockages and interferences in your body, which then enhances energy and allows the body to heal.

What causes blockages? Let's go back to my five core principles of wellness…eating poorly, not exercising, having poor posture, not getting enough sleep and having a bad attitude cause blockages and interferences.

Some basic stressors such as financial issues, relationships, work or school and not managing our time, will cause blockages and interferences. All of these causes don't allow your energy to flow. A good metaphor would be visualizing a river flowing. It's vital, it's energized. Now visualize that the river has a dam. It's blocked. Well our body has many rivers of energy (qi) and what I look for are the areas that are blocked. That's what I am trained to do.

Stressors are the building blocks of this metaphorical dam. If we can learn to become free from these stressors, the dam will crumble and our rivers of energy (qi) will flow freely. With manual therapy, once I find the interference it can be removed or reduced by the therapies we provide.

This is the essence of healing... allowing your energy to flow freely.

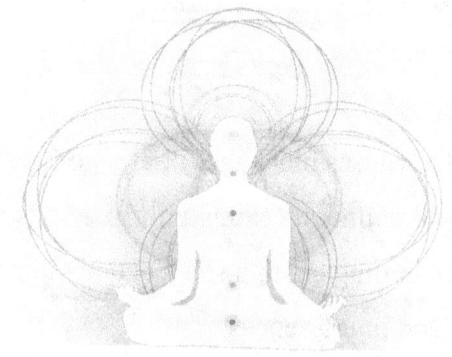

"BounceBackAbility" and Flexibility

This is one of my favorite words. I think we all have periods of time when we feel pain, feel depressed, feel tired or feel that things aren't going in the right direction. As far as I'm concerned it's okay and normal to feel.

It's not okay to stay in that place for prolonged periods of time. Feel what you feel, accept it and learn to let it go, to release it. Being knocked down is fine. How quickly you get up and bounce back is the key.

Another one of my favorite words is "next"… move on. You can learn from what just happened but you can't change it.

The way to have bouncebackability is to have resiliency…. physically, chemically and emotionally. The better your posture, the more fit you are, the more open your attitude is and the healthier your diet, the more flexible you will be.

Pain does not emanate from your physical being alone. It almost always includes a nutritional and emotional component.

I believe good posture and getting enough sleep enhances flexibility.

I believe eating healthy foods enhances flexibility.

I believe having a loving, caring, giving attitude enhances flexibility.

All of these lead us to a place of bouncebackability.

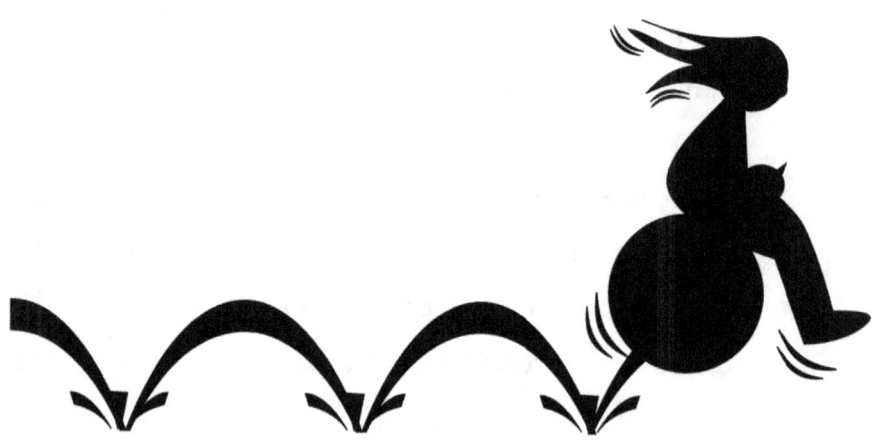

The Triad of Health

One of the foundational elements of health and wellness is the physical, chemical and emotional components all working together in harmony.

As you can see from this diagram each one touches the other.

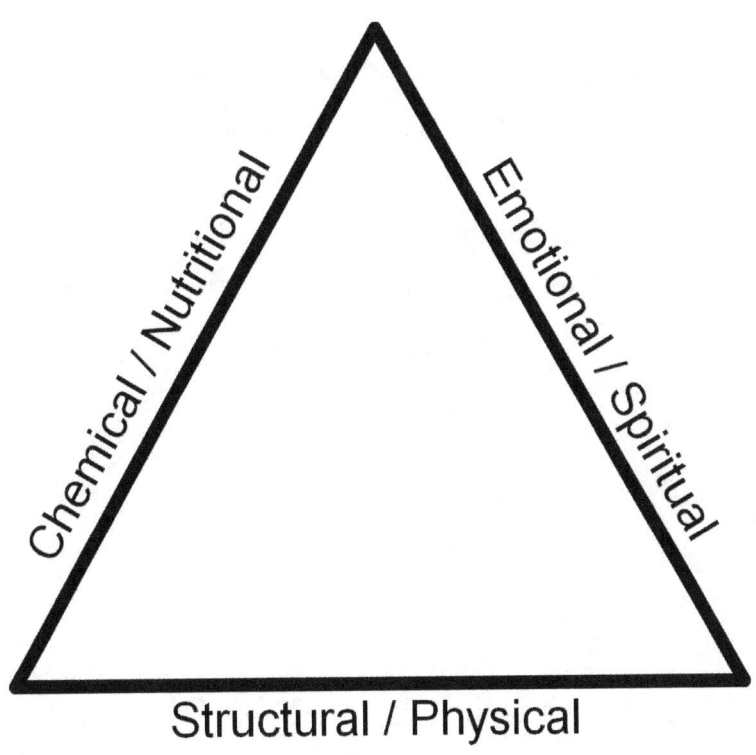

Whatever is going on emotionally and spiritually in your life affects you chemically and physically.

Whatever is going on chemically and nutritionally in your life affects you emotionally and physically.

Whatever is going on physically and structurally in your life affects you emotionally and chemically.

I hope this helps you understand that your physical pain isn't merely caused by physical circumstances.

Getting healthier and well takes time, patience, change and action. Be kind to yourself, take it slow. Even a 1% change each week can yield a 100% change in 2 years.

What Kind Of Stress Do You Have?

Physical / Structural

- Overweight
- No Exercise
- Poor Posture
- Incorrect Exercise
- Not Enough Sleep
- Improper Lifting
- Poor Ergonomics
- Auto Accidents
- Falls
- Chronic Illness

Emotional / Spiritual

- Family
- Relationships
- Finances
- Work
- Time Constraints
- Worry
- Fear
- Guilt
- Anger
- Depression

Nutritional / Chemical

- Poor Diet
- Processed Foods
- Sugar / Soda
- Caffeine
- Alcohol
- Electromagnetic Radiation
- Preservatives
- OTC / Prescription Drugs
- Nicotine
- How you eat: rushed, in the car, on the subway, etc.

Peruse This Chart To Identify Which Areas You Need To Improve Upon

The Best Way to Start Your Day

An affirmation is positive self-talk. So many people say or think to themselves: "I can't, I shouldn't, I don't like this, I don't like that." I have a saying: "You can if you think you can... You can't if you think you can't. "

Negative self-talk (stinkin' thinkin') creates emotional toxicity and tension in your body. I ask my patients to affirm "today is a great day" to themselves as often as they can. They are quite surprised at what a small shift in perspective can do.

One of my favorite affirmations is, "Today is a great day and I have the opportunity to show up as the best me ever." I start my day with an affirmation, and I recommend that my patients do so too.

I also start each day with what I call an "hour of power." It doesn't have to be an hour, it could be fifteen minutes of meditating, relaxing, or setting your mind to visualize the day you want to have.

A lot of people wake up to a loud buzzing alarm clock, push the snooze button a few times and then end up rushing and being behind throughout the day. No wonder they feel tired and stressed!

This creates turbulence in your life, which creates stress in your body. The opposite of turbulence is inner peace, a peace that enables you to take on whatever happens during the day because you can trust and relax through it.

Unfortunately, we have so much turbulence and stress thrown at us in the modern world, that inner peace can be difficult. If you do have inner peace, by appreciating each individual moment, you can better manage the turbulence that goes on every day. That's the goal.

There are so many things that can have a positive impact on your life if you practice them: Affirmations, positive self-talk, optimism, meditation, being loving, being caring, being giving, etc. These states of mind will affect your life in a fantastic way, because you will slowly be releasing blockages in your mind, which then helps the nervous and muscle systems to relax. Love is the antidote.

Your thoughts and beliefs create your reality. Whatever your thoughts are, that's your reality. If your thoughts are kind, giving and loving, you see that reality in a world full of stress around you. On the other hand, if you have thoughts of fear, anxiety and judgment that can place you in that kind of reality. It's your choice.

It's All About Choices

People have to make choices all day, every day. The course of their lives is determined by these small choices made day in and day out.

I tell my patients that they can choose wellness over illness. Of course, the action and preventative steps that you take are imperative (five core principles), but the choice is theirs.

I prefer to start my day with affirmative, positive, loving thoughts. This seems like a better choice for me to create the kind of day I want to have. I want to have a positive, loving day, so I seed those thoughts into my mind.

Do I do it every day? No. Do I get upset and beat myself up if I miss doing it? Sometimes! But I try not to.

It's not about being perfect, because none of us are, but it's about what choices we can make to propel our lives and bodies in the direction we want. We can be excellent, we can be outstanding, but we can't be perfect. Perfection creates rigidity. This book is all about flexibility, not rigidity.

I mentioned before how important it can be to live in the present. To really focus on where you are and what you're doing in the moment. Mindfulness is enriching for your mental well being.

Another small choice that makes an enormous difference is exercise. So many of my patients would never have pain or need my services if they would just exercise more regularly. This is a choice you can make that will determine how well your body performs throughout your life.

I sometimes ask my patients "If you only had one car that had to last your entire life, how would you treat it?" They tell me that they would get checkups, change the oil, fill it with good gas and use it properly. I tell them that they only have one body, so why not make similar choices?

Exercise, drink water, eat healthy foods, and don't overdo anything that can harm your body.

It's not about being perfect, but simply making better incremental choices. Some people will go overboard, and think they have to live in a bubble. I don't believe that. I believe in moderation, not deprivation.

Do you have wine with dinner? Sure, why not. Do you have a bottle of whiskey for lunch? You probably shouldn't.

Do you get enough sleep? Most of my patients don't. We live in the city that "never sleeps," but it can take a toll on both your mental and physical health.

If you aren't getting seven to nine hours of sleep each night, ask yourself why not? Are you worried about something either in the past or future? How can you let it go? Will focusing on the moment help? Maybe you're awake because you're doing something else. What is so important? Is that late-night TV show that important? If it is, then record it and watch it during the day or on the weekend.

What kinds of foods are you eating? If most of what you eat is on the run, or out of a box, that's probably creating more stress in your body. I like to teach my patients to eat things that were alive at some point. It's not that you have to be a super vegan, but just don't eat a bowl of sugar-laden cardboard for breakfast...or ever!

Dehydration is a major problem for people, and easily remedied by drinking water throughout the day to stay hydrated and energized. I always recommend squeezing fresh lemon into your glass of water. What healthy choices will you make today?

Suppression or Expression

Sometimes it's easy to have all of your emotions and stresses bottled up inside of you. One great way to relieve that pressure and heal is a method called, "Expression."

Instead of "suppressing" all of the negative, let's "express" it. We all have some darkness in our lives (negative) but we also have light (positive). Try to have your light shine through.

All of the alternative approaches to healing are about expression, the release of tension and allowing energy to flow. In life, or in a relationship, you want to express yourself, communicate, open up...even be vulnerable. It's a much healthier place to be.

We're in a society where people take lots of medication to suppress and mask symptoms. An alternative way to heal is to express the symptoms, and follow the clues backwards to find the cause of the problem.

You want to express and get it out, which is what I do with hands-on manual therapy. That's what acupuncture, massage, yoga, and meditation do. We find the imbalances and then we relieve the pressure by letting it out.

That's what communication does; it gets it out. We want to have "the negative, toxic stuff" out of our lives from the inside out, rather than suppressing it further and further, where it gets deeper and deeper.

My peers, the baby boomer generation, are in their forties, fifties, and sixties and have been suppressing everything for years. Now their bodies are paying a price.

We have to get it out. We have to let go. We have to allow, we have to surrender. We have to relax. I practice in New York City where people "push and shove and go," but if you push on that door it will never open.

If you take a step back, you might see that there's a sign on the door that says, "Pull," and then you can easily just allow and gently pull the door open or let someone else push it from the other side. It doesn't always have to be a struggle.

Doors open all around us, but we have to be open too, opening our lives, our minds and our bodies. When Chiropractors talk about having good posture, we describe it as being "open" and "free."

Performers open up to their audiences, and they often talk about being in the "flow" of things. Some performers say that when they open up, they feel free to do their work easily.

Very often we become closed down inside, and we shut off so much of our power and strength. That adds emotional and physical stress. It weighs on our shoulders, creates poor posture, and that's why so many people have chronic and acute back problems, as well as various other health challenges.

Many years of holding onto the pressure of life weighs us down and creates poor posture which can lead to serious health complications.

Isn't it better to open up and express, rather than shut down and suppress?

If you're reading this right now and your posture is poor, sit up straight! Take a deep breath, relax, walk, stand and be proud. You deserve it!

Patience

True healing takes time but relief can sometimes be immediate. We are in a quick-fix society looking for instant results overnight.

Fortunately, chiropractic or medication can provide relief. The real question is, what are you looking for?

I ask every patient if they want temporary relief (helps the symptom but doesn't address the cause), maximum correction (correct the cause of the problem for maximum stability) or wellness care (long term preventive care).

Wellness care takes patience and commitment. Helping patients feel symptomatically better has been the easier part of my journey in the health care field.

Helping patients change and improve their lifestyles to pursue wellness is a much bigger challenge.

I get frustrated because sometimes I want patients to change their habits more than they do. It always comes back to what choices we make and how proactive you want to be regarding your health.

For those patients who exercise regularly and go to the gym, it took time to build up muscle strength and stamina. For those who are pursuing the wellness lifestyle it takes time to break down the barriers and walls that have been built up for years.

Be patient. Be kind to yourself. Everything in life that is worthwhile takes time.

What Is an Alkaline Diet versus an Acidic Diet?

We talk endlessly about weight loss in our society because statistics show seventy percent of Americans are overweight or obese. Understanding the difference between alkaline and acidic foods can be a very effective way to eat healthier, which in turn, leads to natural weight loss.

The poor diet that many Americans consume consists of meat, white bread, sugars, butter, mayonnaise, ketchup, soda, sweetened juices and canned and processed foods. These are considered acidic foods.

Foods that are alkaline are healthy. They consist of whole grains and greens such as broccoli, asparagus, brussel sprouts, peas, spinach, cucumber (to name a few). Fruits, such as lemon and lime, tomato, avocado, banana, coconut, are the most alkaline. Oils such as salmon, almonds, olive oil, flax seed and sunflower oil are also very alkaline, and of course drinking lots of water, while squeezing fresh lemon in it. A more extensive chart at the end of this chapter gives you more choices of what's alkaline and what's acidic.

There are four things I discuss with my patients regarding diet:

1) Eat foods without labels. Foods that are in boxes and cans include chemical additives, colorings and preservatives that we usually can't even pronounce. If we can't pronounce it, I don't think we should be eating it.

2) Eat foods that are the colors of the rainbow (ROYGBIV), red for tomatoes, orange for oranges, yellow for bananas, green for broccoli…you get the idea.

3) When you shop in a supermarket, buy foods that are on the perimeter of the store, where many of the healthier foods are.

4) Calories are not an issue if you eat whole, natural organic foods.

We've all seen the commercial for the Eveready battery. It's an alkaline battery and has a lot of energy. That's what alkaline foods do for us. They energize us.

On the other hand, think of a battery in a car that's corroded. It's acidic. It's dead, no life, no energy. That's what acidic foods do to us. There is no life, no vitality and no energy.

47

Another example of how detrimental acidic foods are, if a drop of acid is poured on the carpet, it would burn right through the carpet. When you eat acidic foods it works in a similar fashion by metaphorically slowly eating away at your body.

Since our bodies have an innate inborn intelligence and have a great ability to heal, we produce a "buffer' to protect ourselves from the acidic foods. This "buffer" is called…FAT.

The more buffer your body needs, the more fat is produced. Therefore you can't lose fat in a healthy natural manner if you have an acidic diet.

So, hopefully, I have presented a good reason to eat healthy. Instead of being worried about calories, be concerned with eating healthy alkaline foods and the excess weight will come off.

Common Alkaline Foods- Eat These Freely

Vegetables

- Brussel Sprouts
- Peas
- Cucumber
- Cabbage
- Celery
- Garlic
- Spinach
- Chives
- Zucchini
- Cauliflower
- Onion
- Artichokes
- Turnip
- Carrot
- Radish
- Red Beets

Fruits

- Lemon
- Lime
- Tomato
- Avocado
- Banana
- Cherries
- Coconut
- Watermelon
- Grapefruit
- Cantaloupe
- Dates
- Plums
- Cranberries
- Blueberries
- Strawberries
- Oranges
- Tangerines
- Peach
- Pineapple
- Pear

Grains

- Spelt
- Lentils
- Tofu
- Lima Beans
- Soy Beans
- Brown Rice
- Wheat
- Quinoa
- Buckwheat
- Amaranth
- Kamut

Nuts & Seeds

- Almonds
- Brazil Nuts
- Hazel Nuts
- Walnuts
- Pine Nuts
- Pumpkin Seeds
- Sunflower Seeds
- Sesame Seeds
- Caraway Seeds

Fats

- Olive Oil
- Flax Seed Oil
- Evening Primrose Oil
- Sunflower Oil
- Coconut Oil

Fish

- Salmon
- Halibut
- Sea Bass

Common Acidic Foods- Eat These Foods in Moderation or Sparingly

Meat, Poultry, Fish
- Red Meat
- Pork
- Oysters
- Clams
- Liver
- Organ Meats
- Eggs
- Chicken
- Veal
- Swordfish

Milk Products
- Homogenized Milk
- American Cheese
- Processed Cheeses

Bread
- White Bread
- White Pasta

Beverages
- Liquor
- Wine
- Beer
- Coffee
- Sweetend Juice

Fats
- Margarine
- Corn Oil
- Butter

Sweets
- Artificial Sweeteners
- White Sugar
- Fructose

Misc.
- Ketchup
- Mayonnaise
- Canned Foods
- Processed Foods
- Microwave Foods

Balance Comes in Threes

I've talked a lot about flexibility and bouncebackability but there is a third component of health called Balance. I have found that things come in groups of 3 to complete a cycle of balance.

- There are 3 categories of exercise:

    Stretching

    Strengthening

    Cardiovascular

- There are 3 primary stressors:

    Physical

    Emotional

    Nutritional

- There are 3 major food groups:

    Proteins

    Carbohydrates

    Fats

- There are 3 choices regarding how you pursue treatment for many back related conditions:

    Drugs

    Surgery

    Therapy

- There are three foundational pillars that I recommend to obtain better posture:

  > Core strengthening

  > Postural consciousness and standing proud

  > Enhance flexibility of hamstrings and gluteal muscles

- There are 3 techniques that I utilize in my practice to restore flexibility and balance:

  > Chiropractic manipulative therapy

  > Trigger point massage

  > Physiotherapy

I can go on and on but I think you get the idea. Be aware of these packages of three to make better health care choices, which will ultimately lead to a more balanced life.

One last metaphor about threes:

When we point our index finger as if we are blaming someone or something else, remember there are three fingers pointing back at you. This goes back to my saying "If you don't go within....you go without". Start looking inside yourself for more answers to better health.

What Are The Causes of Back Pain?

When I was trained in Chiropractic school, we learned that traumas, falls and accidents were the primary cause of back pain. After 34 years in practice, I continue to see a growing trend of emotional stressors such as relationship issues, finances, work or school and time management much more often the cause of many patients' back problems.

How do I know this? When I sit down during a consultation with a patient, I ask "What do you think caused your back pain?" and the response is usually "I didn't do anything!" After 90% of my patients said this, I realized the impact of how emotional stress manifests in our physical bodies.

Only 10% of patients told me they either lifted something, fell or had an injury. This is pretty shocking to me but there is one other intangible: poor posture! Sitting at a computer for eight to twelve hours per day, which many of my patients do, in combination with the emotional stressors seem to be the true cause of back pain.

This brings us back to asking: "**Why** am I having this pain"?

Strategies and Action Steps For A Healthier Spine

When I discuss with patients what their responsibility and commitment needs to be in order to become healthier, I always say "Either you're in the pain or....you're in the pain".

This simply means that you're either in the pain you originally came to my office with, or you're in the pain of trying to change your habits.

Sometimes it can be painful to create new habits such as beginning an exercise or stretching program, changing your eating habits, being more aware of your posture, getting more sleep and maintaining a loving, caring, giving attitude.

Doesn't that sound like my five core principals?

Action Steps- Simplified!

Here is a simplified list of action steps that you can take today in order to have a healthier spine:

Walk more

Be conscious of your posture

Stretch or take yoga classes

Breathe in your nose and out your mouth

Smile

Drink a lot of water with lemon

Eat more fruits, vegetables and whole grains

Be more loving, kind, caring and giving

Have an attitude of gratitude

Let go

Get more sleep

Write down your to-do list before bedtime

Exercises - Keep it Simple

For those of you that go to a gym or health club consistently, I applaud you. I believe only about fifteen percent of Americans are actually committed to physical exercise at least three to five times per week.

For the other eighty-five percent I try to keep it simple so exercise can be easy even if you don't go to the gym.

We're going to explore three basic areas of stretching that I believe are essential to having a flexible and healthful body.

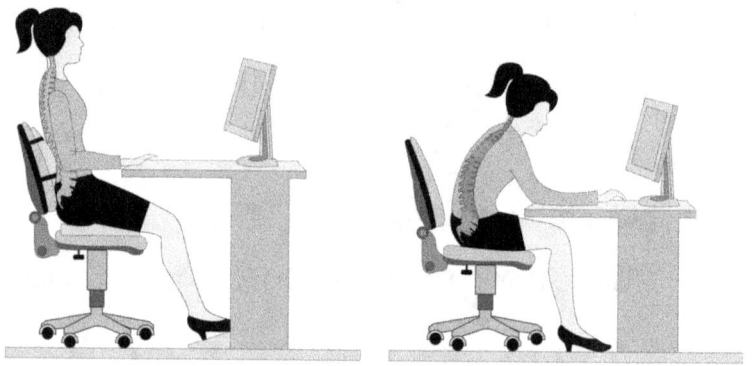

Posture

1) Let's start with posture. I believe posture is the most important exercise, because I call it the exercise of consciousness.

Just by being more aware of our posture (sitting, lying or standing) better overall health is the end result.

Standing with your arms spread out and opening the chest while you breathe deeply is a fantastic way to recharge and refresh your body. It also helps to keep your spine aligned and good posture.

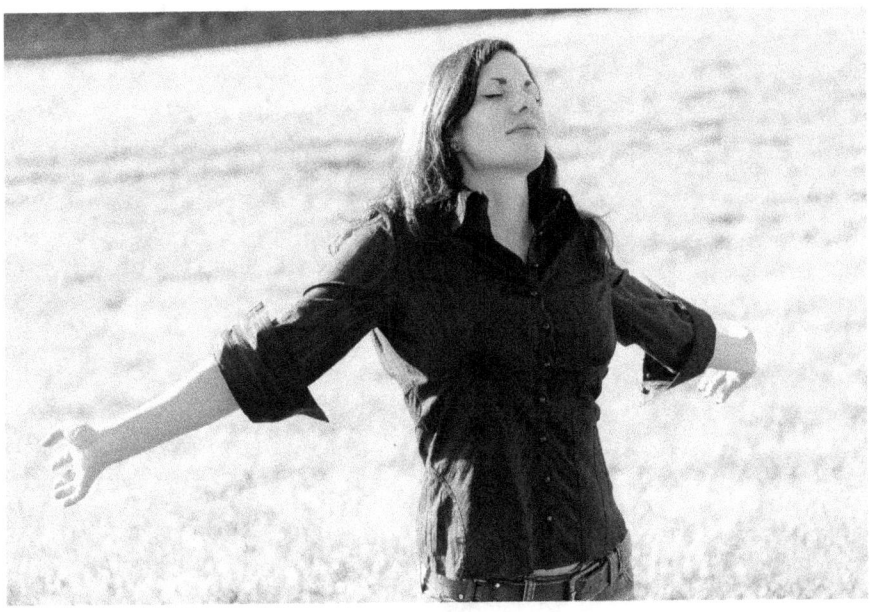

Plank Exercise

2) In addition to posture, enhancing core strength is imperative. Even if you are overweight you can improve your core strength by doing the plank exercise every day.

Just hold a push up position on your forearms for as long as you can. If you do this daily, you can get the support and strength you need in the front part of your body. (abdominals and pectorals)

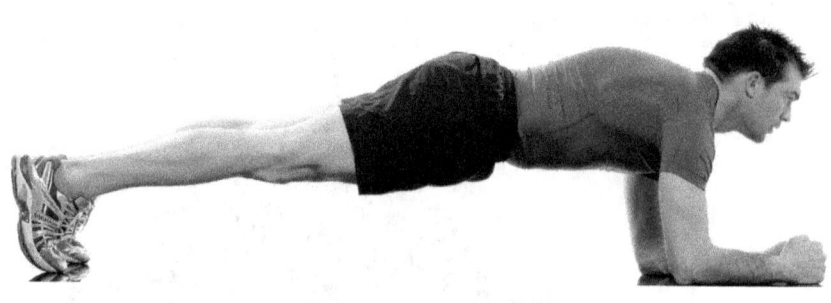

Lower Body

3) The third key component to exercise is flexibility of your hamstring, gluteal and spinal muscles. These are muscles in the back part of your body that need to be stretched. (See the photos below)

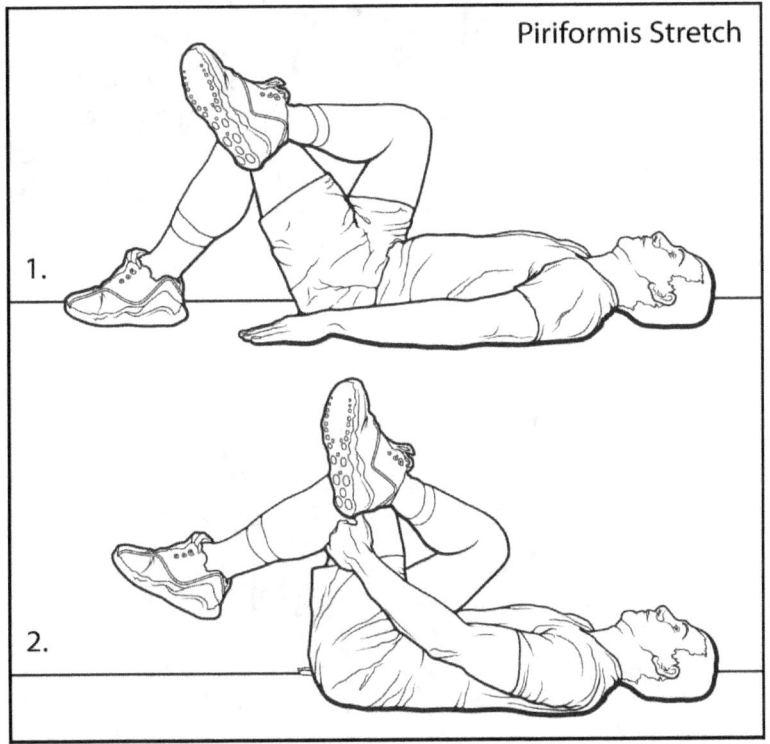

Piriformis Stretch

1.

2.

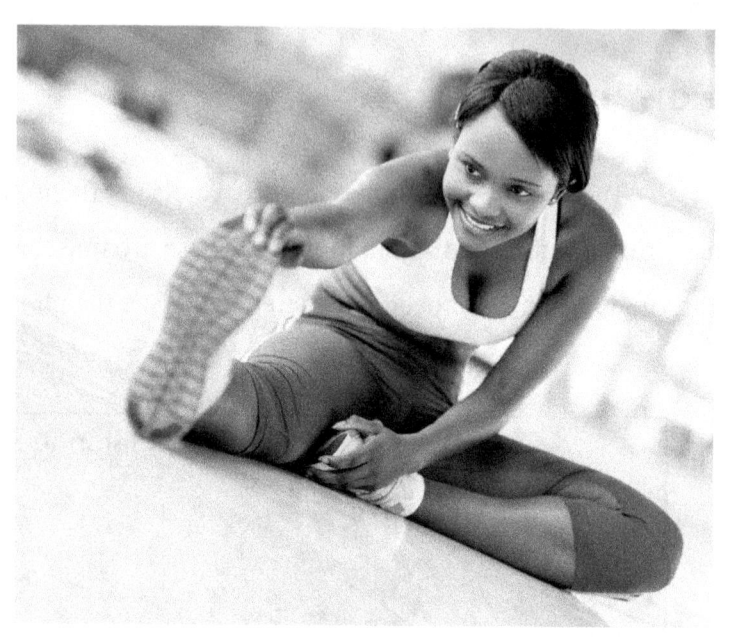

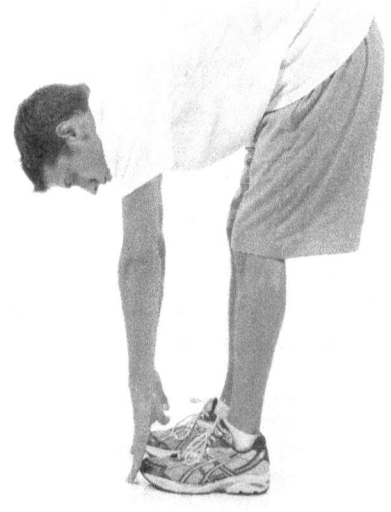

Your Immune System

If we are going to talk about wellness, we must discuss the immune system. It's our bodies' defense system. When the immune system is strong, we are healthy and well. When our immune system is compromised we are vulnerable which is when we get sick or break down.

We've been taught that we get sick from the germs around us, our kids, coworkers, etc. The reality is that germs are always around us (we can't even see them) in elevators, on doorknobs, with food handlers, in bathrooms, everywhere! We blame others for us getting sick (I caught this cold from my…)

The fact is we get sick and our body breaks down when our own immune system has been compromised. What weakens our immune system, you ask. We have to go back to my five core principals and I'll bet all five are not being adhered to.

When you don't sleep, don't eat well, don't exercise, have poor posture and don't have a loving attitude, your immune system breaks down.

How do you explain a classroom setting where one of the children is sick, coughing and sneezing? I will admit maybe half of the class gets sick, but what about the other half that still attends class. They were exposed to the same germs. Why are they perfectly well? In my opinion, it is a result of their stronger immune system.

How do you explain when the pollen count is high, some people suffer with allergy symptoms and others are fine. We are all breathing the same air with the same pollen. Those with a stronger immune system don't suffer with pollen or other allergies.

Keep your immune system strong by implementing the five core principals of wellness.

Interrupting Patterns = Changing Habits

Even though I'm a Chiropractor, I like to call myself a "pattern interrupter". What I'm trying to accomplish with every patient that walks into my office is to begin the process of shifting the responsibility of getting healthy back to the patient. I believe all health care providers are here to help, but the more you work on you, the chances of you being healthier increase greatly.

As we've discussed, to make lifestyle changes we must begin by integrating the five core principals of wellness into our everyday life. Small shifts from poor posture to improved posture or beginning a stretching program become major pattern interrupters.

The manual therapy that I provide also interrupts patterns. By utilizing trigger point therapy I release the tension that has settled into the musculature. Once these blockages and interferences are removed or reduced, new healthier patterns begin to emerge.

If you are satisfied with where your health is, keep doing what you've been doing. If you are striving for better health, take a closer look at your habits and take some action steps today.

Relationships

The most important relationship you can have is with who? The answer is, with **yourself**. Health and wellness is about you working on you, growing you and making better health care decisions. This is a life long journey and process of being committed to living a healthy lifestyle.

Once you begin building your relationship with yourself, your self-esteem and confidence grows, which leads you to making better choices regarding your health.

Just as I talk about being physically flexible, it is so important to be emotionally resilient. If one can practice forgiveness, non-judgment of others, and kindness, wonderful things can happen in life.

Self-esteem and self-confidence go hand in hand with our posture. Simply put, good posture comes from strong self-esteem and poor posture can come from low self-esteem. It's called state management, or in other words, how is your emotional state impacting your physical state.

This is all part of becoming more whole. The more whole we are, the more we attract whole people into our lives. The needier we are, the more we attract that into our lives.

Healthy relationships come from you, not to you.

Be the **CHANGE** you wish to see in the **WORLD**

Patient Affirmations

Here is an affirmation that I've used for many years to start my day:

Today is a great day and I have the opportunity to show up as the best me ever!

I am an irresistible magnet with the absolute power to attract into my life everything that I desire. My life is a huge success!

I am committed to constant and never-ending personal improvement, and I take massive action steps to create the future as I want it. I will do whatever it takes to become the winner I know I can be.

My beliefs create my reality! I choose robust health, abundant wealth, constant happiness and eternal love. I attract, heal, and positively influence the lives of people in my community. I think big thoughts, relish small pleasures and handle all setbacks gracefully.

I give thanks for the opportunity to serve humanity and I willingly accept the rewards being sent to me by an abundant universe. I am deeply grateful for all I create and receive. My life is now in total balance.

Using affirmations on a daily basis is one of the simplest and easiest action steps you can take to get what you want, and you should know that affirmations done on a daily basis can and will change your self-image.

Affirmations are positive statements that stimulate your mind with an attitude of expectancy! Affirmations control the thoughts that you think. Affirmations are your opportunity to condition yourself to be exactly who you want to be.

Here are some personal affirmations that you can carry with you to read and say aloud, with enthusiasm:

- I can do anything I want to do!
- I am doing what I love to do!
- I know whatever I need to know for my wellbeing, success, joy and fulfillment
- I am approaching my ideal weight, easily, naturally and permanently!
- I feel strong, confident and worthy of success!
- I am magnetized to abundant health!
- I am a happy person!
- I love to laugh and enjoy life!
- I see the good in every situation!
- I see abundance and opportunity at every turn!
- I take full responsibility for me!
- I am a good saver of money!
- I love getting out of debt!
- I am financially prosperous!

- I am rich!
- I am successful in everything I do!
- I am generous, kind, supportive and compassionate!
- I am serene, calm, peaceful and without stress!
- I give more than I receive!
- I have value as a person!
- I am professionally very competent!
- I am a magnet for all good things!
- I love to give!
- I am a minister of encouragement, a master of comfort to people, a communicator extraordinaire!
- I attract money into my life!
- My potential is unlimited!
- I can have it all!
- I am worthy of my success!
- I am a success and it is easy and comfortable to be so!
- I am my dream come true!
- I am wonderful!
- I am confident!
- I am self-assured!
- I am unique!
- I am worthy!
- I am wisdom!

- I am truth!
- I am beauty!
- I am wealth!
- I am harmony!
- I am courage!
- I am excitement!
- I am health!
- I am abundance!
- I am destiny!
- I am peace!
- I am successful. I am success. I am love!
- YES, I CAN! YES, I WILL! YES, I AM!

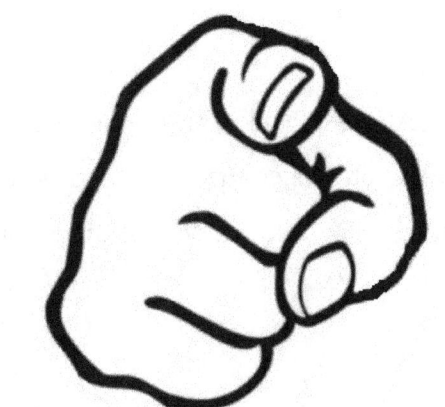

WHO IS THE AWESOMEST?
YOU ARE!

Patient Testimonials

"I have been a patient of Dr. Angrist's for close to 10 years, which proves my experience has been wonderful. The bed-side manner, courtesy and professionalism I receive is always authentic and genuine. My stress level management and overall wellbeing stems from the care I receive at Angrist Chiropractic. My regular adjustments have become an aid in how to deal with day to day obstacles. This care truly gives me more energy and drive to face challenges head on. I encourage and promote holistic healing, especially when I've experienced the best. Thank you."

–C.Z. 2012

"Dr. Angrist, thanks for treating me so well last week. I was a stranger and you treated me like a long time client. I didn't think I'd get through the week, and you changed that! I'm grateful!"

–D.P. 2012

"I remember in 2099, when I was first introduced to Dr. Angrist by co-worker, that I had a lot of pain and pressure in my head and neck. I've seen lots of chiropractors over the years for this condition and had eventually stopped seeing all of them. During this particular bad time, Dr. Angrist was nice enough to fit me in as a new patient as soon as I could make it into his office, which I thought was very nice of him. Dr. Angrist is the only doctor who took the time to listen to my ailments and offer to help me not only with treatments, but to explain why the body behaves in certain ways and how changes must be made to eliminate the everyday stresses of our lives.

Because of a very stressful work environment, it is not always easy to follow Dr. Angrist's easy and calming attitude for life. But he never loses faith in you and continues to treat your body and speak to your spirit. Both must be paying close attention because I have seen a noticeable difference. I'm very glad that my co-worker put me in touch with Dr. Angrist. He has made a difference in the management of pain, which was a constant companion, and is only too happy to share his wisdom on managing life's sometimes turbulent roads. It's a pleasure to have a doctor who would rather treat the root of the problem rather than suggest surgery."

–A.G. 2012

"I have been Dr. Angrist's patient for eight months. I started going to Dr. Angrist because I moved from Phoenix, Arizona and was no longer able to get adjustments from my father, who has been my chiropractor for my entire life. My back pain has been minimized and I feel like Dr. Angrist is more than just my chiropractor. He always gives me advice on staying healthy and is somewhat of a father figure since my father is so far away. I always look forward to relaxing, de-stressing, and feeling better when I go in for my appointments. Thanks Dr. Angrist & Team!"

– J.R. 2012

"I've been seeing Dr. Angrist for around 4 months and he has helped me considerably. I used to suffer from overwhelming back pain, which often prevented me from doing the things I love to do. With his help, my pain has decreased significantly. The practice's interest in wellness care has also been inspiring; I find I'm more active, eating better and paying attention to my body more than I used to. Overall, this has been a hugely positive experience and I'm grateful for the help I've received from this center."

– A.H.2012

"I have been going to Dr. Angrist for almost 20 years. He always makes me feel much better physically as well as mentally. You always feel that he really cares about you."–Patient 2011

"There are no words to say how Dr. Angrist has helped me, mentally, physically, internally. I have been seeing Dr. Angrist for over 3 years and it has not been easy for me. I have had a few setbacks and some relapses that really scared me. Dr. Angrist has told me that stress also plays a part in one's body healing. I used to depend on a back brace and a cane to get around, and I was in so much pain all the time. But by going to see Dr. Angrist, my rehabilitation has improved my movement and flexibility. I do have bad days, but my body is able to spring back. He really has helped me deal with my injury. I feel I'm making great results!"

– A.P. 2012

"My entire body feels better as a result of the care you have given my back, and I find myself taking better care of my body than I did before I started getting adjustments from you. I always look forward to my visit." – Patient 2011

"Dear Dr. Angrist, You have helped me through what has been a very difficult and painful journey and you have literally improved the quality of my life. I strongly believe God sends "special people" into our lives to take care of us...thank you so much for all that you do and for your words of wisdom."

–Patient 2011

"You have made me so much more aware of me and life itself. I learned to think more positive and act on it which in turn made me healthier".

– Patient 2011

"As an avid tennis player, I have come to rely on Dr. Angrist's diagnostic and therapeutic abilities to repair the sporadic injuries that the sport incurs. He has never failed to correctly diagnose the site of the problem and alleviate the pain. My wife has chronic back and sciatic nerve condition, Dr. Angrist has almost a magical ability to relieve her suffering during her acute episodes."

– Patient 2011

"Doc you are truly one of the most precious blessings in my life. Thank you for being my doctor, nutritionist, therapist and friend. May God continue to bless you with wisdom, good health, a caring and peaceful nature and a loving nature."

–Patient 2011

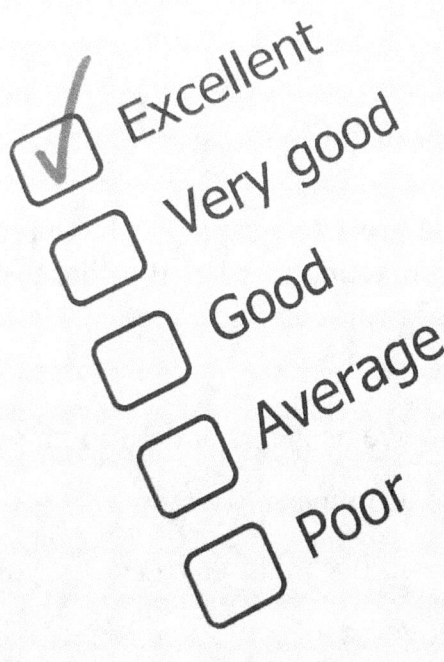

"Dr. Arnieisms"

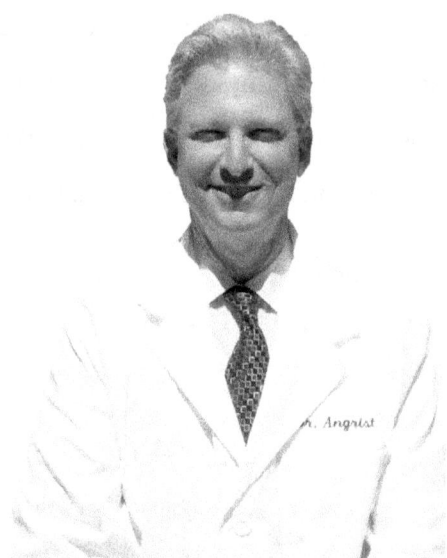

These are a few sayings I have picked up during my 34 years in practice that I really like to repeat. I hope you find them as useful as I do.

- God gave us 2 ears and 1 mouth so we can listen twice as much as we talk.

- You can if you think you can…you can't if you think you can't.

- The most important things in life…aren't things. Family, health and happiness are.

- Have an attitude of gratitude
- Don't have stinkin' thinkin'
- Stop blaming and be accountable
- Motion affects emotion
- Your body doesn't lie…all you need to do is listen to it.
- Your belief creates your reality.
- Do you have a job, career, or a calling?
- Do you think paying for alternative care is a cost or an investment in your health?
- The past is history, the future is a mystery and the present is a gift…that why it's called the present
- If you don't go within…you go without.
- Most back problems are not life threatening…just quality of life threatening.
- Wellness is not about a product or service…It's about your lifestyle choices.
- Giving is good, but forgiving is better

- Life should be like a candle burning bright until the end, then it should just flicker and go out...not flicker for months or years.

- One of my favorite words...NEXT

- Just maybe...your health challenge is lifestyle related.

- The universal antidote is...LOVE

- All we need is a sliver of light to remove the darkness.

- Eat foods without labels

- To reach your goals ask yourself four questions

    1) What do I want?

    2) Why do I want it?

    3) By when am I going to get it?

    4) What actions do I need to take to get it?

- When it rains and puddles form, what do adults do? They walk around the puddle. What do kids do... they walk right through the puddles...be a kid again.

- The mind is like a parachute... it only works when it's open.

- There are two great days in a person's life... the day you are born, and the day you find out why.

- It's not where you go…it's who you are with.

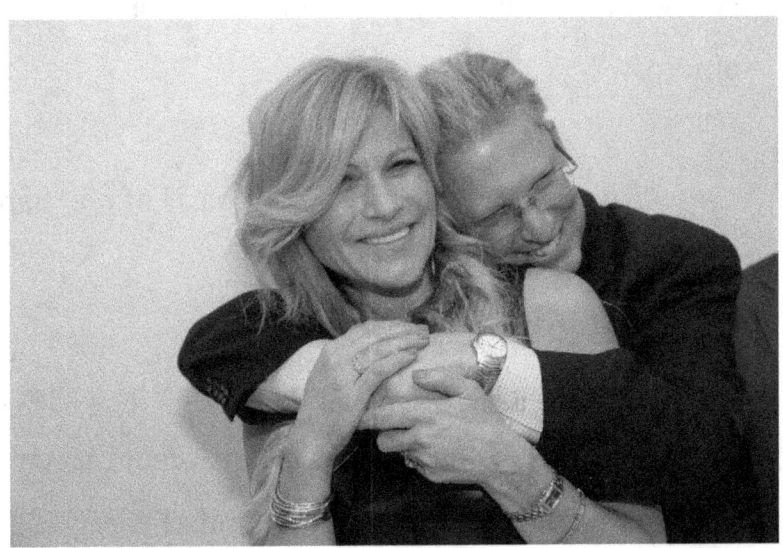

Thich Nhat Hanh quotes:

"Peace is Every Step"

"Our appointment with life is in the present moment. If we do not have peace and joy right now, when will we have peace and joy – tomorrow, or after tomorrow?"

"The absence of anger is the basis of real happiness, the basis of love and compassion."

"When anger is born in us, we can be aware that anger is an energy in us, and we can accept that energy in order to transform it into another kind of energy."

"If we know how to accept our anger, we already have some peace and joy. Gradually we can transform anger completely into peace, love and understanding."

"Do not maintain anger or hatred. Learn to penetrate and transform then while they are still seeds in your consciousness. As soon as anger or hatred arises, turn your attention to your breathing in order to see and understand the nature of your anger or hatred and the nature of the persons who have caused your anger or hatred."

"Learn and practice non-attachment form views in order to be open to receive others' viewpoints. Truth is found in life and not merely in conceptual knowledge. Be ready to learn throughout your entire life and to observe reality in yourself and in the world at all times."

"Do not mistreat your body. Learn to handle it with respect. Do not look on your body as only an instrument."

Personal Stories from Dr. Angrist

I. Love, The Universal Antidote

One of my favorite stories deals with my one on one doctor-patient relationships. Being trained as a chiropractor, the practice of chiropractic is geared towards treating patients using the power of hands on manual therapy. The power of touch has performed wonders for millions of people worldwide for centuries. But what I think is more powerful is the story of love.

I truly believe that if we can come from a higher place of love, caring, giving and being nonjudgmental we can resolve many of the physical ailments in our society. I continue on a daily basis to teach, preach and coach the philosophy of love and letting go. To learn to surrender, open up and relinquish control is the precursor to better health.

If we could just be more patient and allow our body to heal, rather than interfering with the healing process, we can be so much healthier. Emotions such as fear, anger, negativity, ego and even perfectionism get the better of us and block the healing process.

We live in a high tech world, but I think we need to get back to more of a high touch approach, in the form of helping and touching others and just being more loving. LOVE is the universal antidote. Love is the light in our lives. We need to have more of it. It's at least worth a conversation. Just think how healthy you can be with more love.

II. Dave Matthews

On a beautiful Sunday afternoon, I was playing golf with my sons Matthew and Jason. I received a phone call from a woman named Hans who was a representative for recording artists in the music industry.

She asked me if I was available to treat Dave Matthews before he performed at Randall's Island that evening. I told her I was playing golf with my boys and I would not be finished until 6pm. She said that was too late and I said, "I'm sorry, I can't make it." and I hung up.

My son Matthew said to me, "Who was that Dad?" I said, "I was just asked to treat Dave Matthews, but I told them I couldn't because I was playing golf with you guys. In order to get to the stadium on time to treat him we would have to leave now and not finish our round of golf." They said, "Dad! Call her back and let's go." I called Hans and told her the situation and she said, "You can bring your sons with you and go backstage to treat Dave Matthews."

We got off the golf course, called my other two sons, Ben and Jon and told them we were picking them up and going to the stadium at Randall's Island so I can treat Dave Matthews.

All four boys were incredibly excited just for this alone until Hans called me back and said she will provide us a police escort to the stadium! They would meet us at the George Washington Bridge and take us through enormous traffic to get to the stadium on time.

They found the whole experience very exciting and we hadn't even gotten there yet. When we did arrive directly to the back stage area, Hans was waiting for us and brought me to Mr. Matthews' room to begin his treatment. She told me my boys would be in the first row and when I was done to go meet them and enjoy the show.

I treated Dave, went to my seat and saw one of the best concerts I had ever seen. My boys were happy and I was thrilled to share this experience with them.

III. Tony Robbins

One of my patients worked for motivational speaker and peak performance coach Tony Robbins. She told me that Tony needed a chiropractor when he is in NY. Tony has a chiropractor everywhere he travels. I began treating him in the 80's when he would have a seminar in NY, usually for 5000+ people.

He was such a believer in chiropractic care. He would have a treatment before, during, and after each day of the conference. If you don't know, Tony is one of the most powerful speakers in the world, and one of his highlights is the "Firewalk."

This is where he has everyone at the seminar be thoroughly trained to walk on hot coals that reach 2000 degrees. This is done in your bare feet. It sounds impossible, dangerous and frightening but he had a method to overcome fear and this was it. One of the greatest experiences in my life was to not only treat Tony, but to walk on these hot coals on a few occasions. The "Firewalk" metaphor is all about if you can do this you can certainly conquer any fear you may have in your everyday life.

I was honored to treat someone who helps so many people, and in a way I felt like I was helping people "Firewalk" too!

IV. Johnny Carson

I had the privilege and honor to treat Johnny Carson when I was an associate doctor in 1979. He came in with a hip problem and was told he probably needed surgery. He was trying an alternative approach to hopefully avoid the surgery.

One of the first things we did with him was watch him walk on the streets on NY. This way we could see exactly what he was feeling and how he was walking. The funny part was as soon as we hit the street every cab driver shouted out, "Hey Johnny" and you know what he did- he shouted back!

He was loved in NY and he loved us back. The evaluation of his hip turned into an entertaining experience I will never forget.

I treated the King of Late Night for a little while, but it became apparent to me that he really needed the surgery. I had a hard time convincing him, but I knew that it was in his best interest for his health to surgical intervention.

After the surgery he was grateful to have his pain relieved, and I was fortunate to have healed one of New York's Legends. For me, that's what 34 years in practice is all about.

Thank You!

Thank you for reading this book. I hope it has inspired you to take more control over your health and find new ways to improve your life and wellness.

After 34 years in practice, I am so grateful for my patients who have allowed me to help guide them towards a better life.

If you know someone who might want to improve their overall wellness, please send them my way or share this book. I love to help new people, and appreciate every opportunity I get to help.

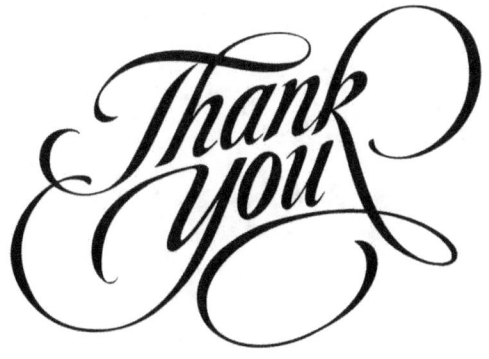

www.AngristChiro.com

www.ingramcontent.com/pod-product-compliance
Lightning Source LLC
Chambersburg PA
CBHW070804290526
45795CB00002B/619